The Book of JOY and Gratitude

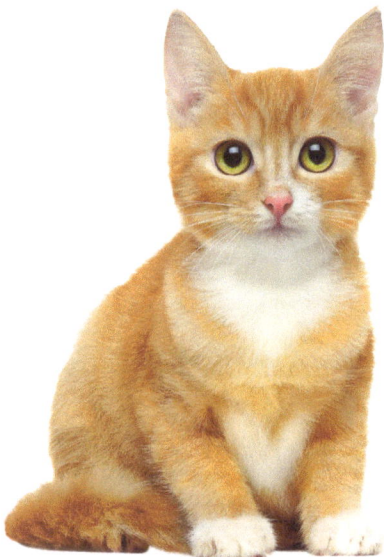

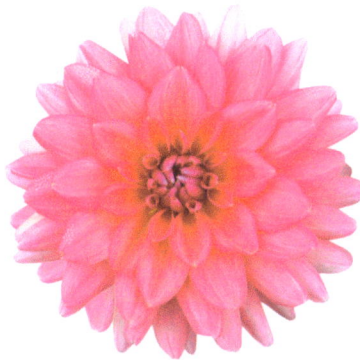

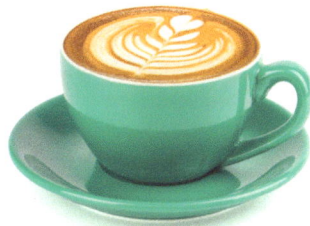

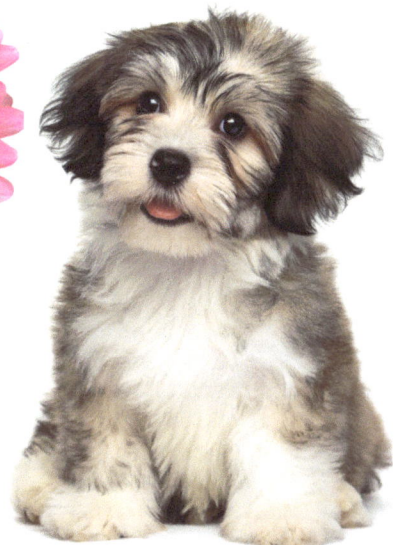

LOMIC BOOKS

The Book of Joy and Gratitude

By Joy Kinnest

ISBN: 978-1-988923-53-6
Lomic Books
Kitchener, Ontario

Copyright

Feedback

Your opinion matters.
Please share your comments and questions about this
book by emailing: jmorend@lomicbooks.com

Lovely Flowers

The simple joy is looking at flowers.

The petals are lovely.

The colors are delightful.

What kind of flower do you like the best?

Welcome to...

The Book of Joy a[...]

Taking the time to be gratef[...]
things in life can help people [...]

In this book, we reflect on bein[...]
everyday gifts such as:

- ✓ **Lovely flowers**
- ✓ **Naps**
- ✓ **Tasty treats**
- ✓ **Doing puzzles**
- ✓ **Television**
- ✓ **And more**

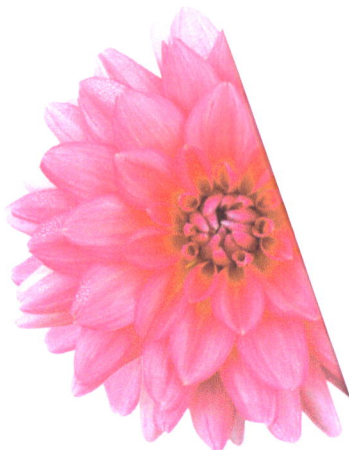

This book can be read two pages at a tim[...]
or simply flipped through to see the lovel[...]
pictures.

No matter how you use this book, we hope [...]
you really enjoy it!

Lovely Flowers

One simple joy is looking at flowers.

The petals are lovely.

The colors are delightful.

What kind of flower do you like the best?

Welcome to...

The Book of Joy and Gratitude

Taking the time to be grateful for the small things in life can help people feel joy.

In this book, we reflect on being grateful for everyday gifts such as:

- ✓ Lovely flowers
- ✓ Naps
- ✓ Tasty treats
- ✓ Doing puzzles
- ✓ Television
- ✓ And more

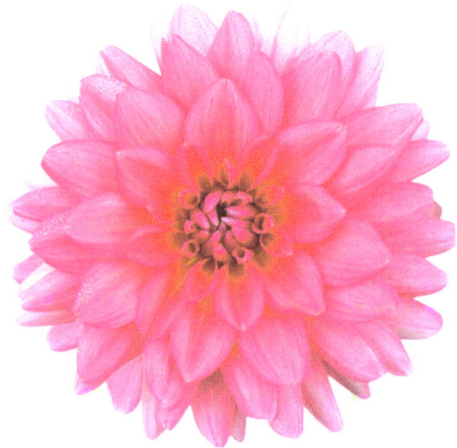

This book can be read two pages at a time, or simply flipped through to see the lovely pictures.

No matter how you use this book, we hope you really enjoy it!

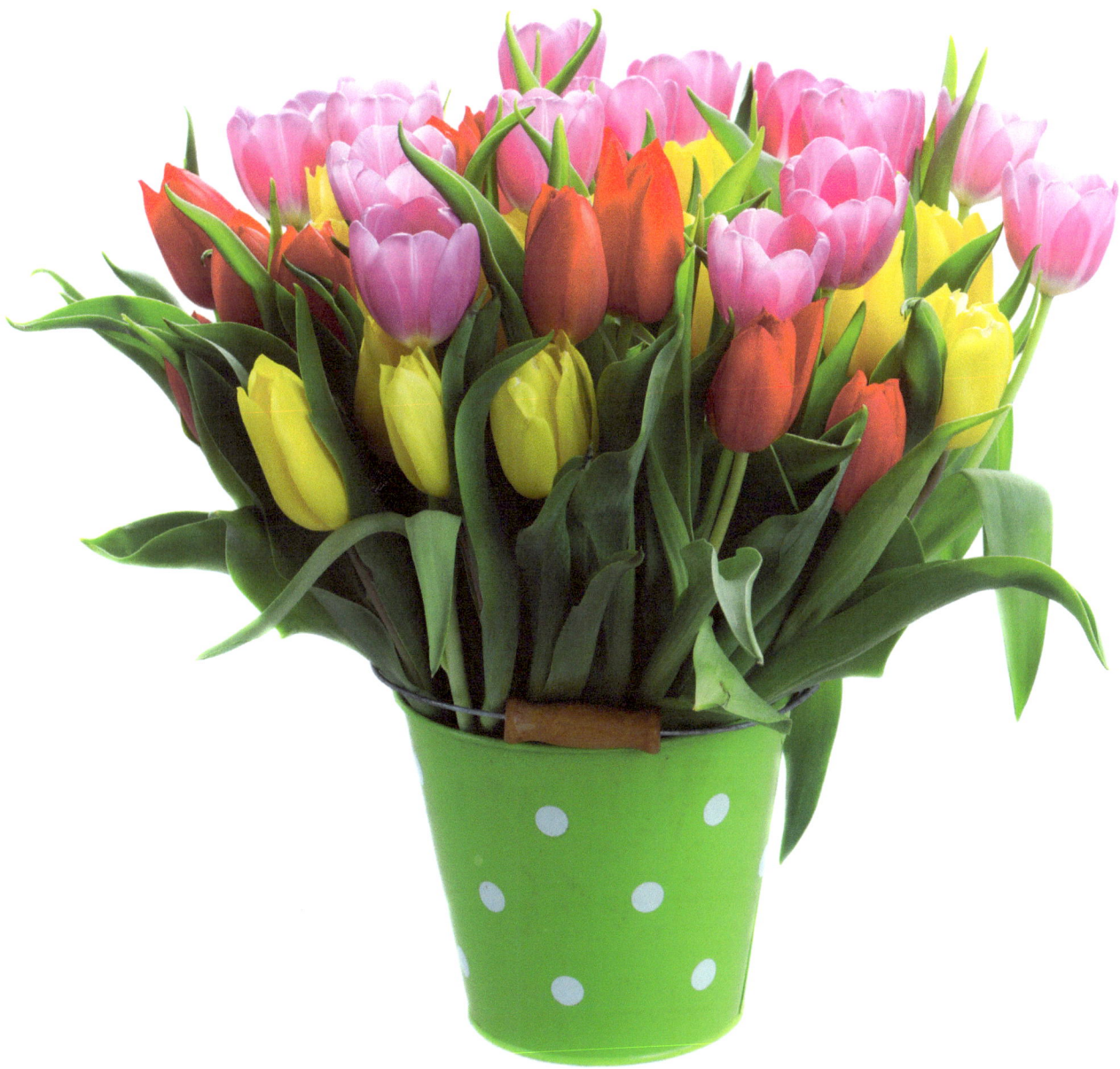

Tea or Coffee

A warm cup of coffee or tea can be a real treat.

There is a lovely smell and a terrific taste.

It can also be a way to relax.

What kind of coffee or tea do you like the best?

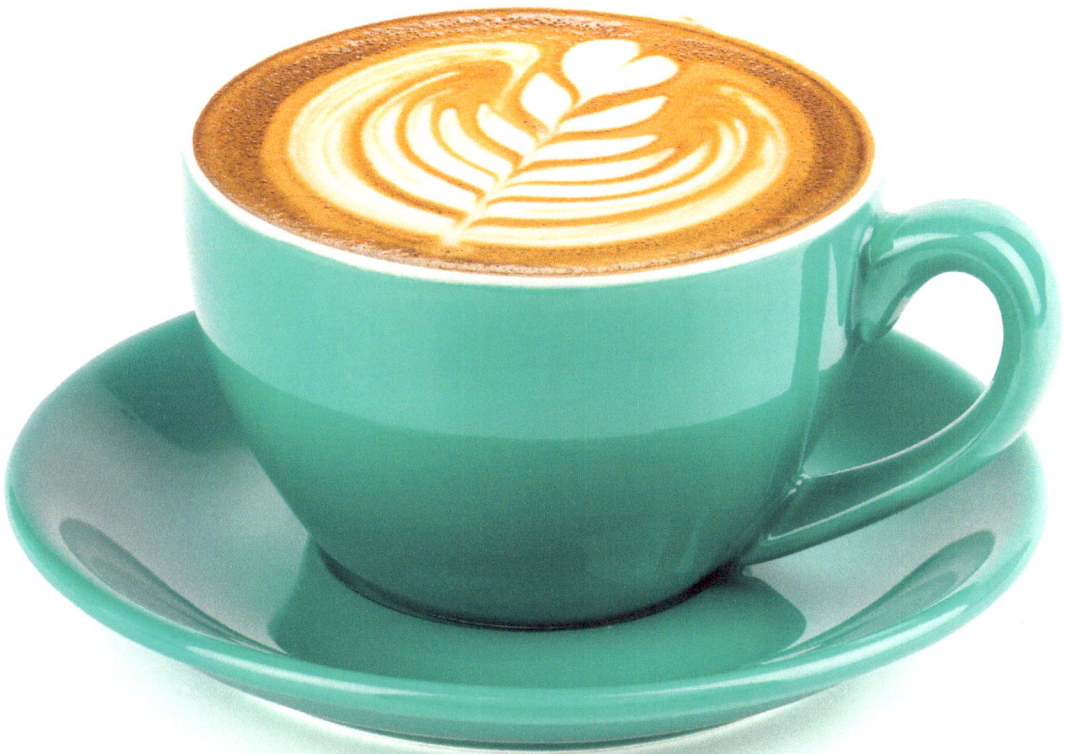

A Nice Nap

To have a lovely rest, when you need it, is one of life's luxuries.

You can take a nap in a chair, on the couch, outside in a hammock, in bed, or any other comfortable location.

Where do you most enjoy taking a nap?

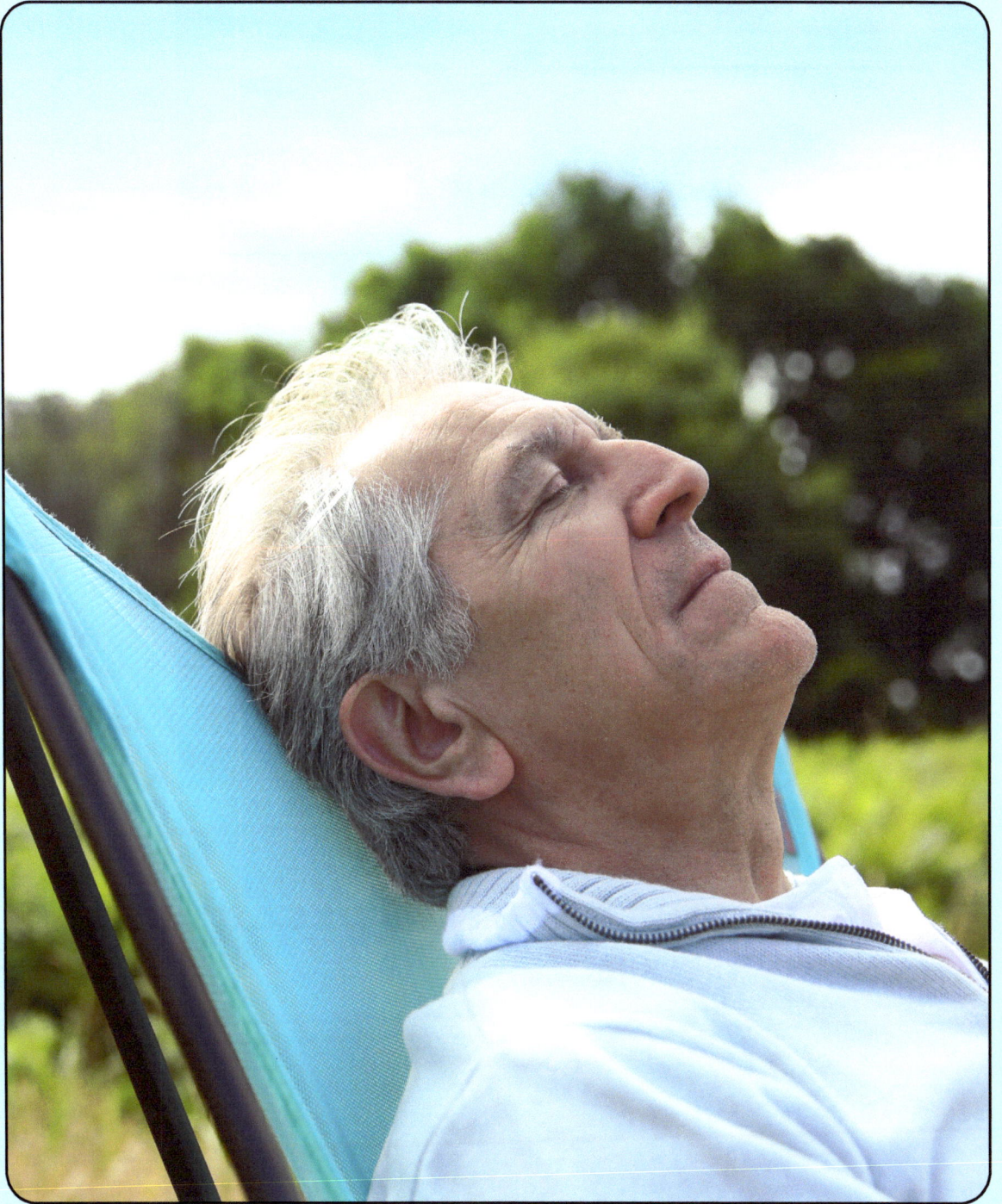

Sweet Treats

A sweet treat can be a joy!

Whether it is candy, cake, donuts or any other delicious treat.

It is easy to be grateful for the taste of a sweet treat.

What is your favorite sweet treat?

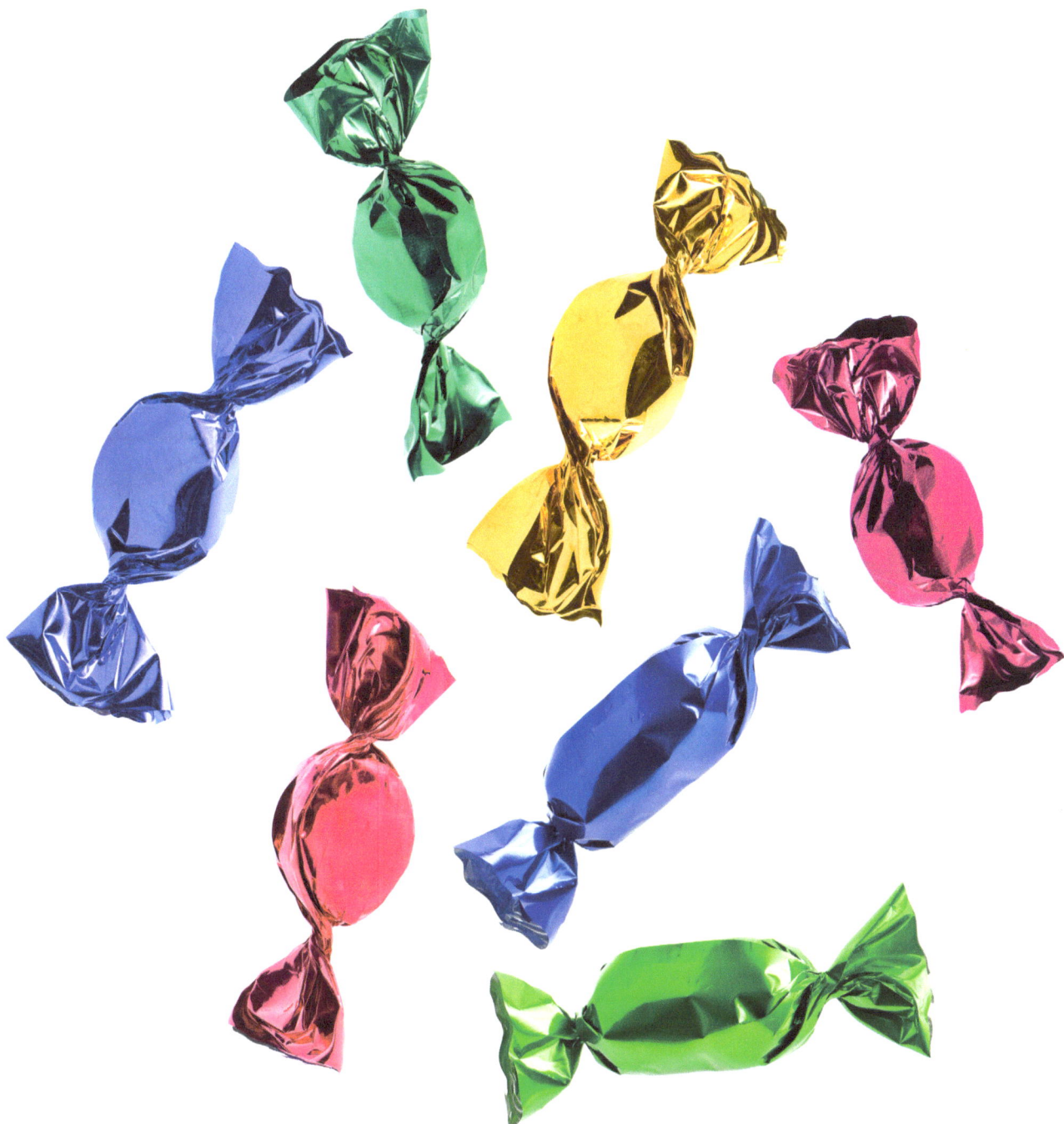

Fun Puzzles

Working on puzzles can be a lot of fun!

You can take your time to think about an answer to a puzzle.

Solving a puzzle feels great!

What is your favorite kind of puzzle?

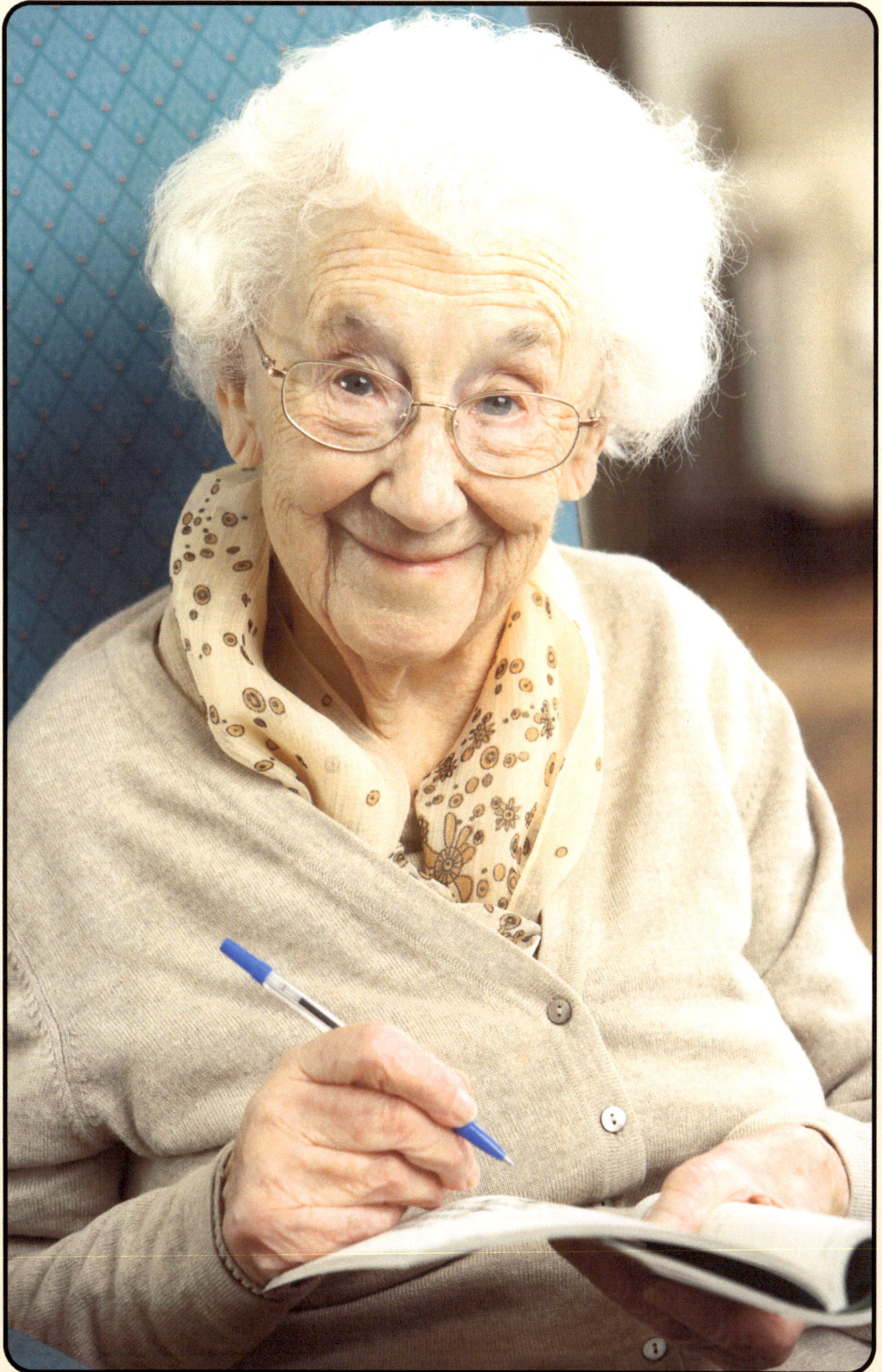

Puppies & Dogs

Puppies and dogs are very adorable.

They can be playful and joyful.

Dogs are often soft, friendly and happy to say hello.

What is your favorite kind of dog?

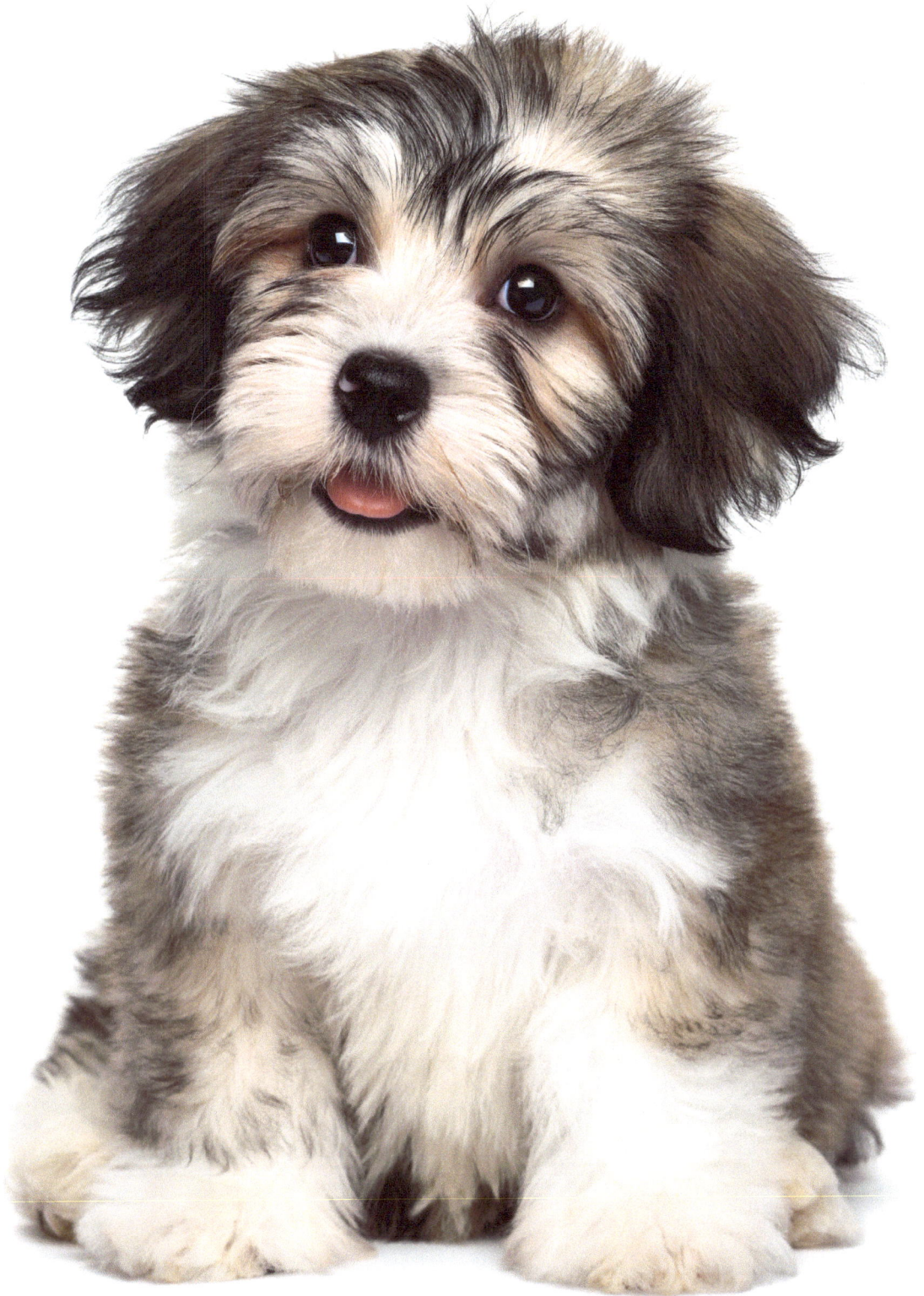

A Nice View

Just looking out the window can be a great experience.

Perhaps you can see a nice blue sky, lush green grass, or lovely trees.

There are so many different things that can make the view out of your window something to be grateful for.

What kind of view do you like the most?

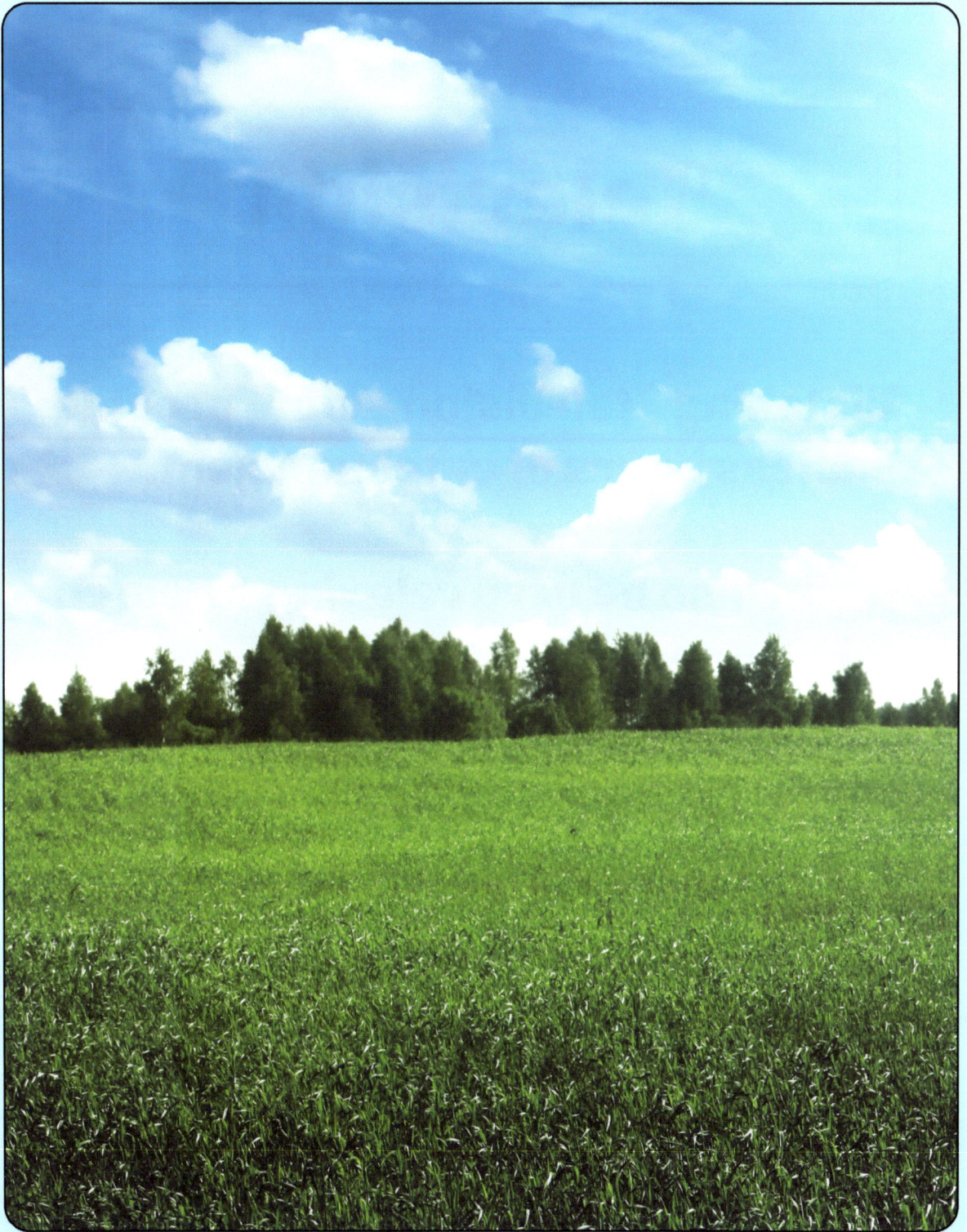

Television

Watching television can provide endless hours of entertainment.

It can also be very relaxing to watch television.

Fun TV shows include comedies, dramas, and game shows.

What is your favorite TV show?

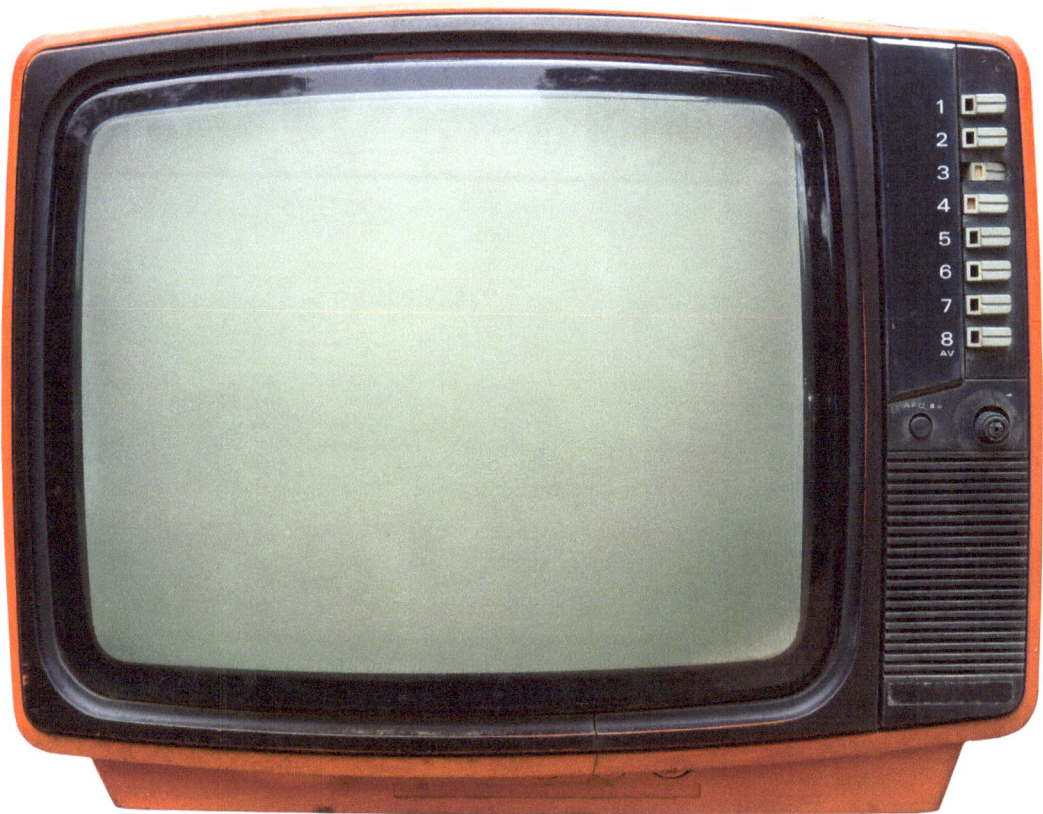

Reading

Reading a book can be a lot of fun.

You can enjoy reading alone, or in a group.

A book's words can take you to places far away, or help you appreciate your life at home.

What is your favorite book?

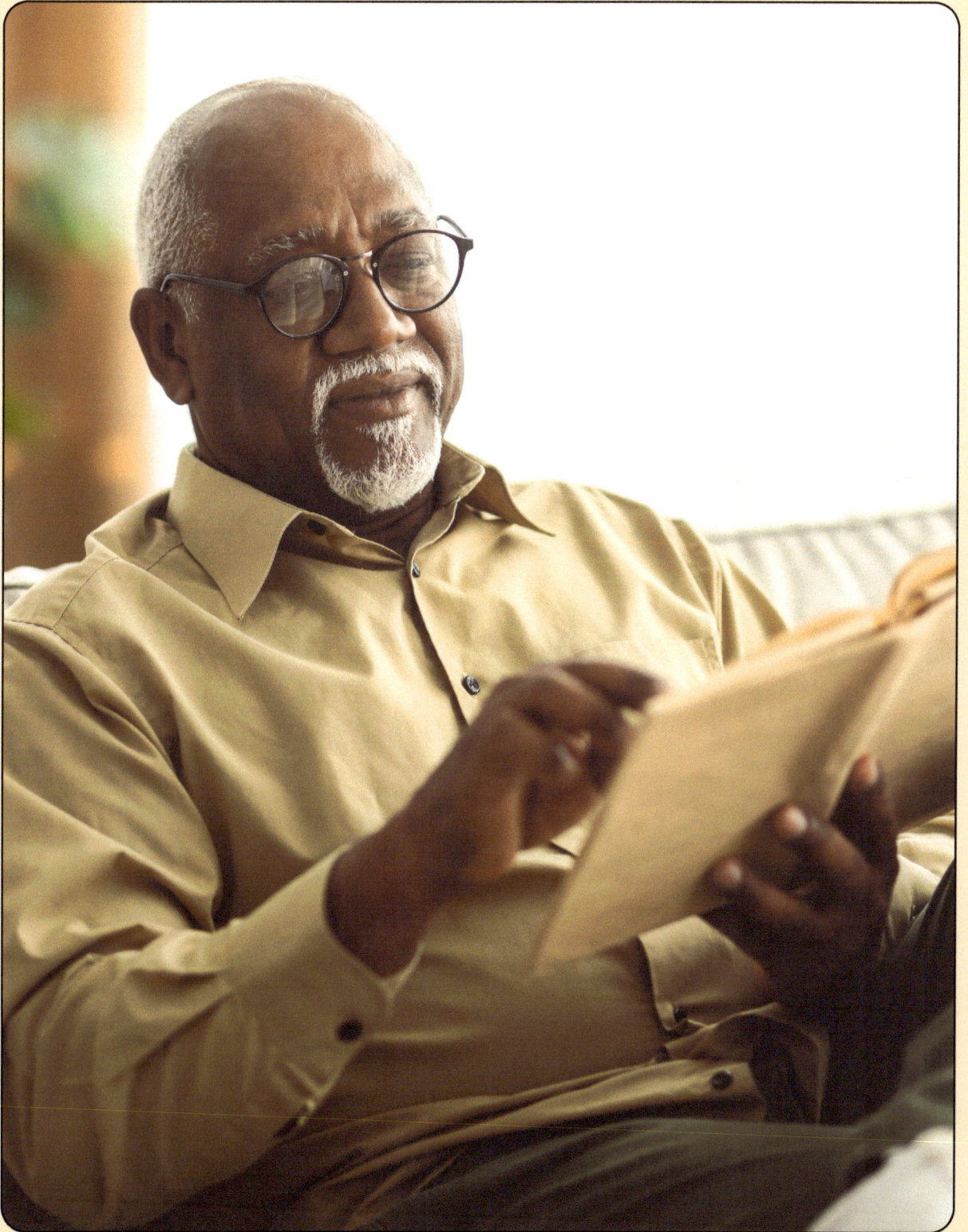

Kittens & Cats

Cats are delightful pets.

Cats are smart and like to play.

Kittens can be adorable, fun and friendly.

What kind of cat do you like best?

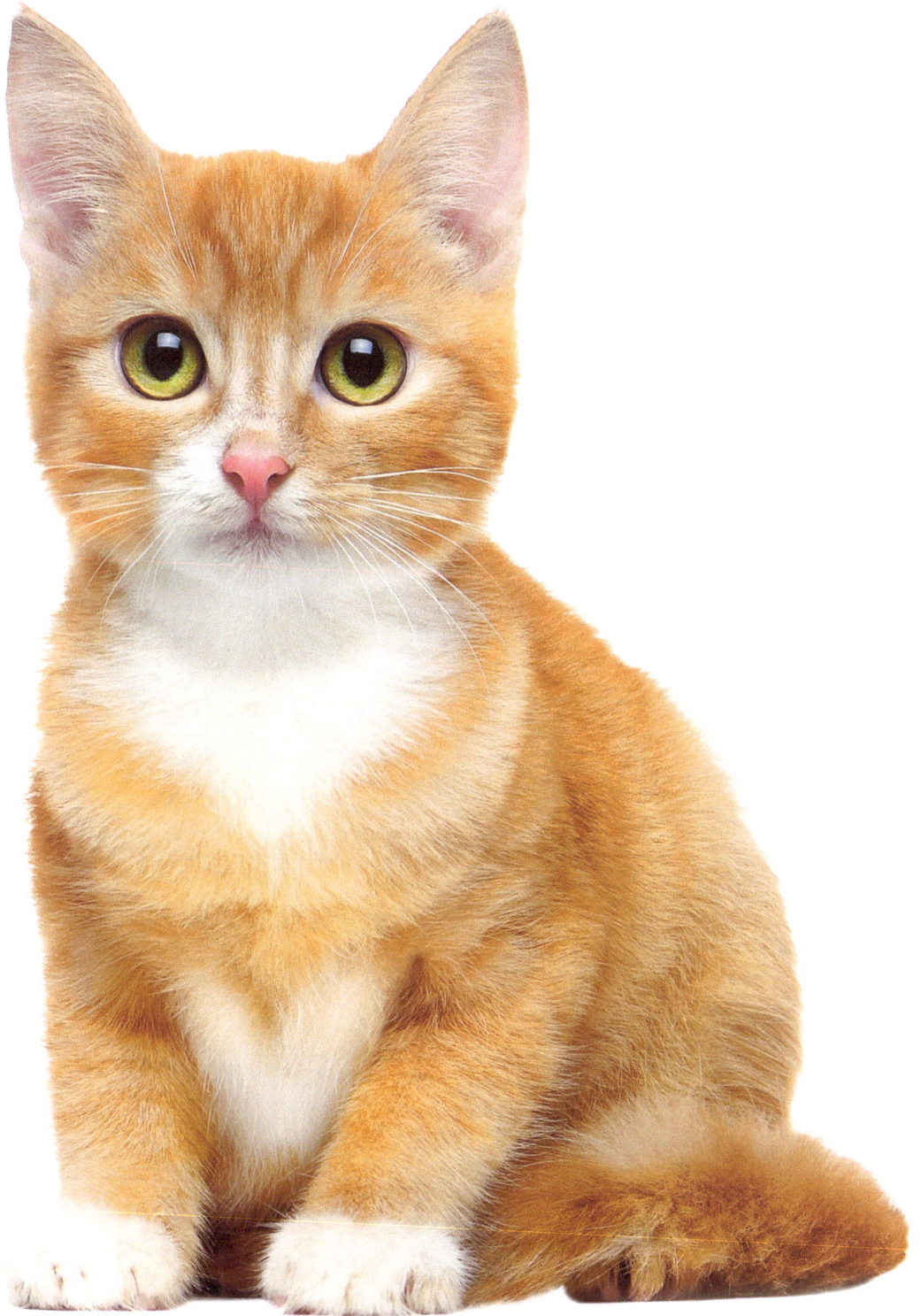

A Phone Call

A phone call from a friend, or a call from family, can be a lovely experience.

It can be a joy to talk to someone you know.

Who do you most like getting a phone call from?

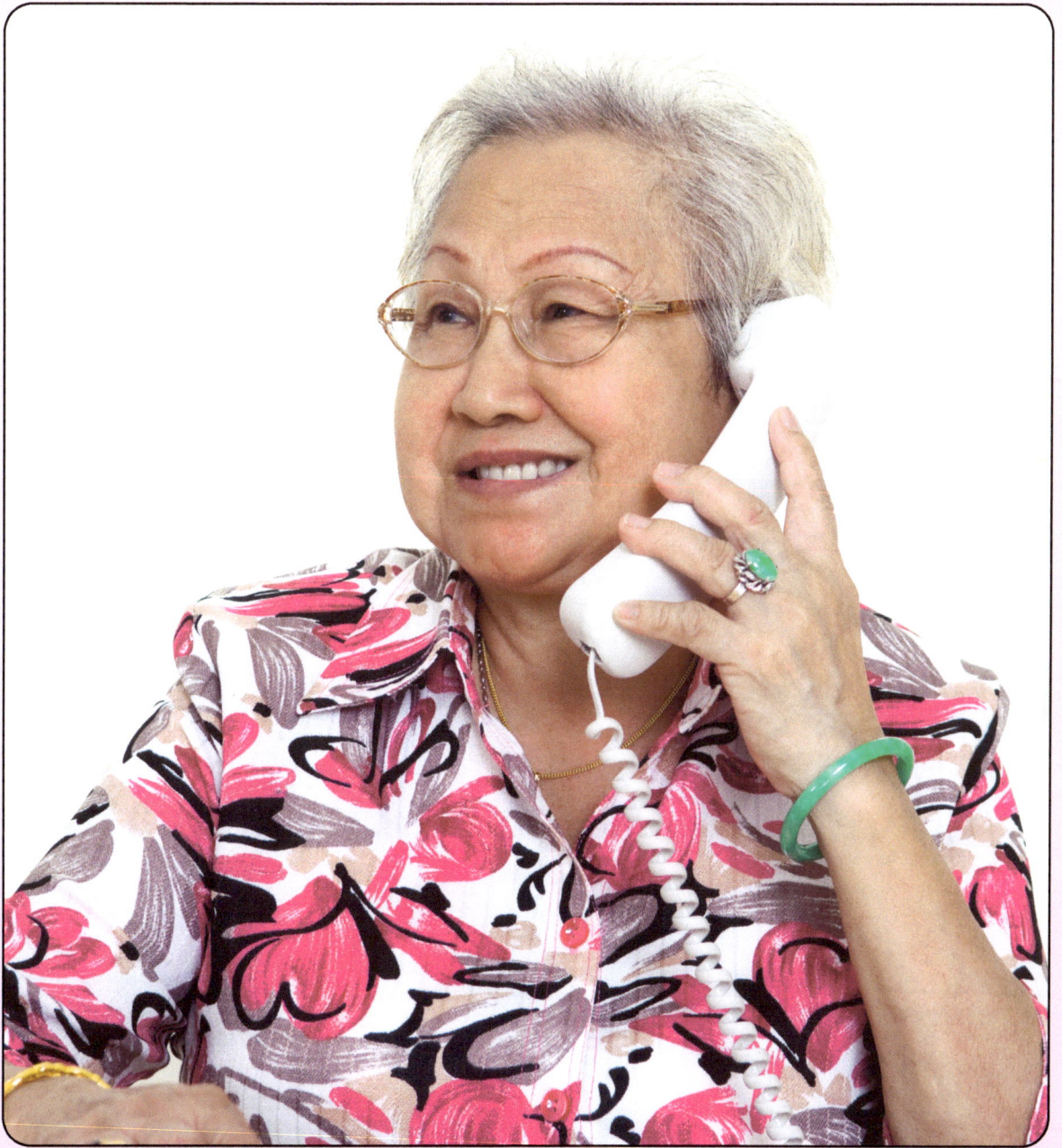

A Salty Snack

A salty snack can be delicious and crunchy.

Salty snacks are can be a real treat when watching a movie, or as an afternoon snack.

What is your favorite salty snack?

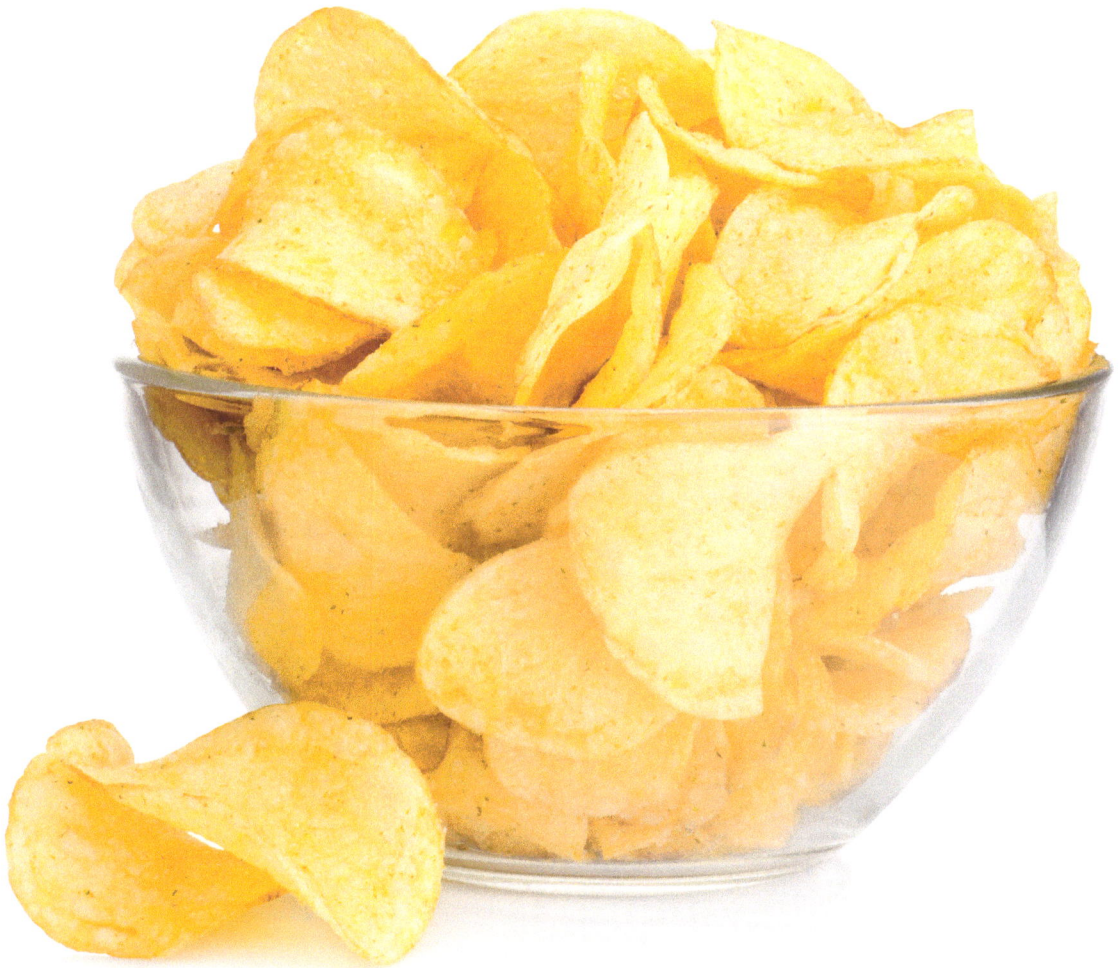

And More...

There are so many other things to enjoy and be grateful for.

You might appreciate a warm blanket, doing crafts, or taking a class.

What else are you grateful for?

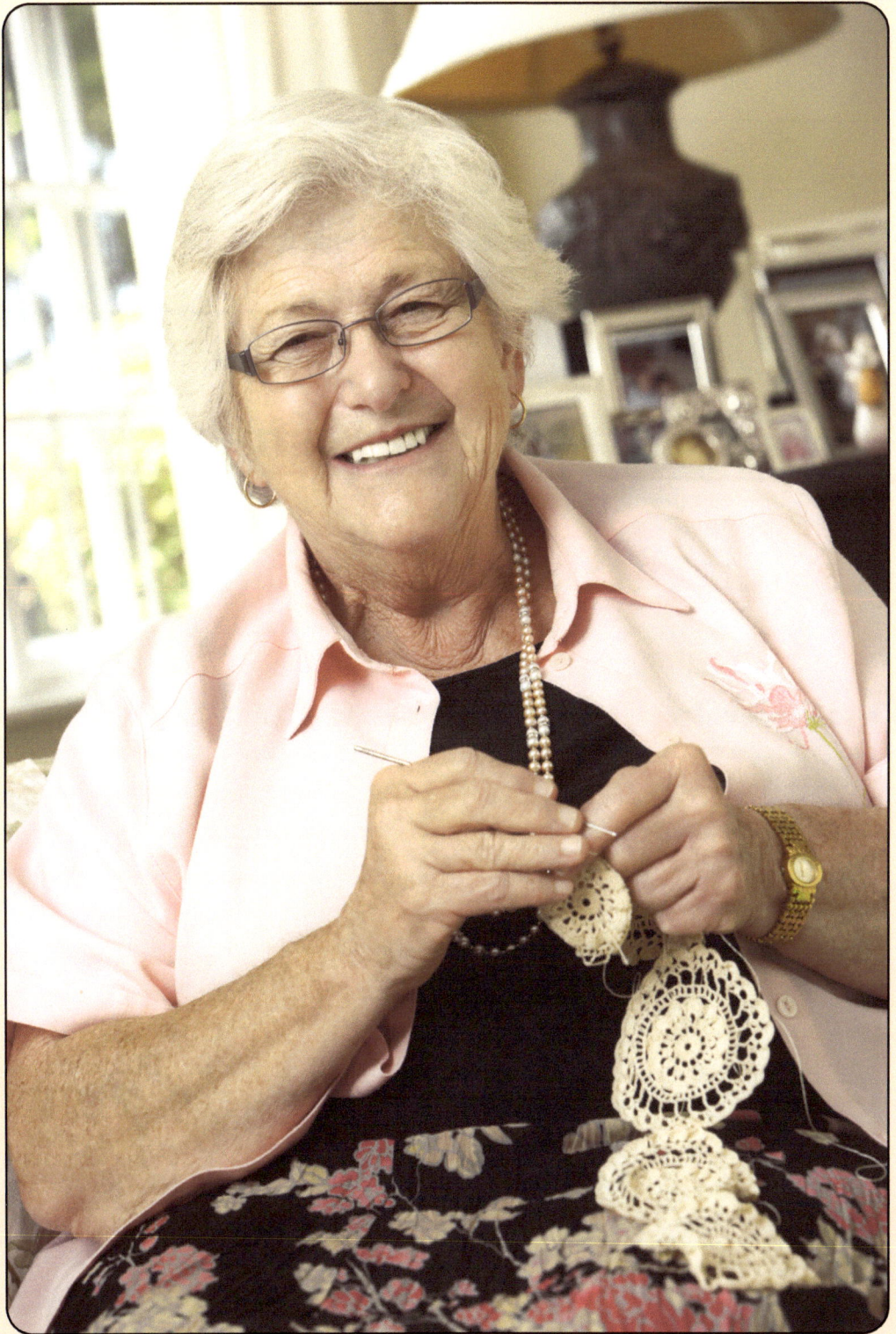

The End

Even endings can be joyful.

A sunset at the end of the day,

The end of an exercise class.

What ending are you grateful for?

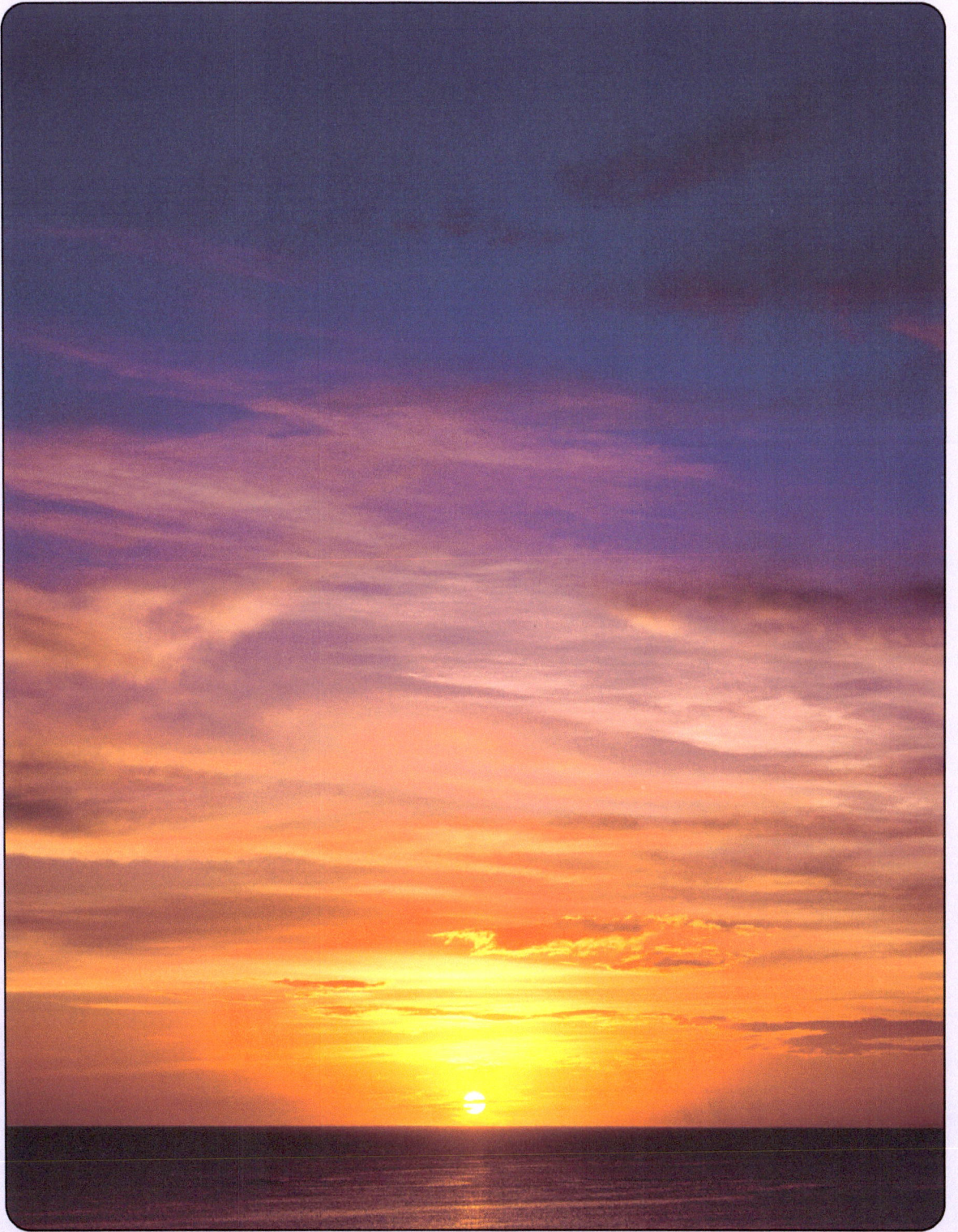

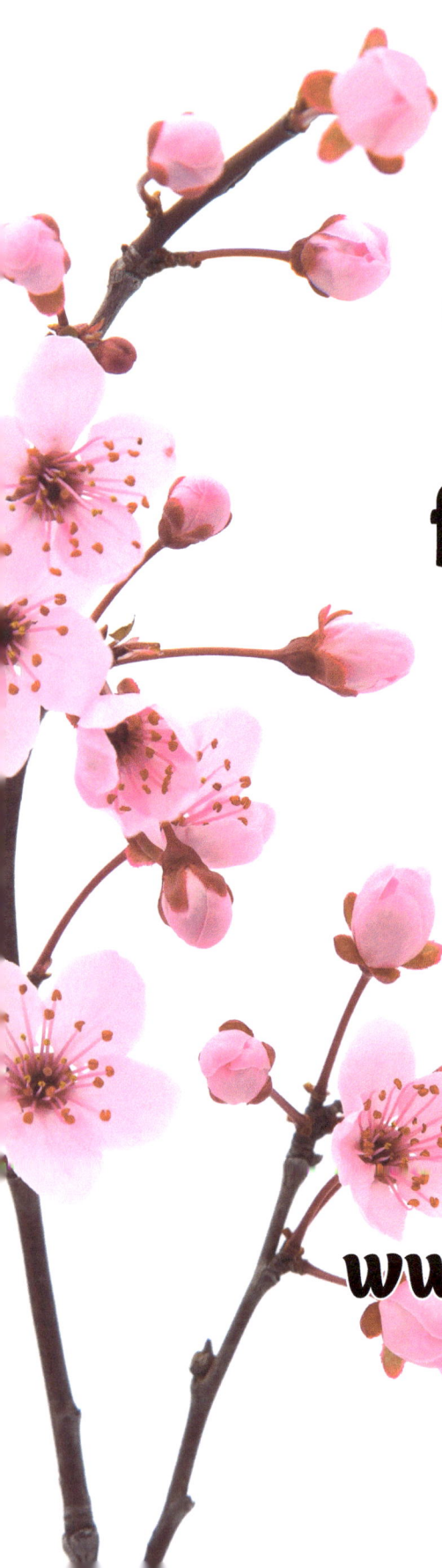

Thank you for reading this book!

For more books check out:

www.lomicbooks.com

www.ingramcontent.com/pod-product-compliance
Lightning Source LLC
Chambersburg PA
CBHW041105050426
42335CB00046B/121